10 Psychology Hacks to Instantly Influence and Persuade Anyone

Get What You Want Now

Jayne Watson

By reading this document, the reader agrees that under no circumstances is the author responsible for any losses, direct or indirect, that are incurred as a result of the use of the information contained within this document, including, but not limited to, errors, omissions, or inaccuracies.

Table of Contents

Introduction

You know your toddler needs their vitamins, yet they refuse to eat their veggies. You have found the perfect house for that lovely newlywed couple, but they are having second thoughts. Everyone needs to persuade someone at some point in their lives, whether to close a sale, feed a child their veggies, or help a loved one change course. It is a highly underestimated skill that is utilized every day by millions of people, yet not talked about enough.

What Persuasion Isn't

We want to think of ourselves as purely logical, objective, decision-makers, and therefore we don't like the idea of someone persuading us. Just think about political campaigns or advertising! But while the word itself may have somewhat of a bad reputation, persuasion is an important skill we should all master. And let me tell you right from the start, persuasion is not about lying or manipulating others, but to help them follow your vision and fully understand your point of view.

Why Should You Learn Persuasion Techniques?

Here are some advantages you'll get by reading this book and applying its tips:

- **Effective Communication**: Develop persuasion skills to articulate your thoughts, ideas, and opinions compellingly and convincingly. It helps you express your message clearly, engagingly, and in a way that resonates with your audience.

- **Building Relationships**: When effectively persuading others, you can foster cooperation, resolve conflicts, and negotiate mutually beneficial outcomes. Persuasion helps you establish trust, credibility, and rapport with others, strengthening your personal and professional connections.

- **Achieving Goals:** Persuasion is often necessary to achieve your desired outcomes in personal or professional settings. It enables you to influence decision-making processes, gain support for your initiatives, and motivate others to take action.

- **Understanding Human Psychology**: By understanding the principles of human psychology that influence decision-making, you'll tailor your persuasive approach to resonate with your audience.

- **Effective Communication Techniques**: The book will guide how to structure your arguments, use storytelling, employ rhetorical devices, and utilize persuasive language to capture attention and sway opinions.

- **Building Trust and Rapport**: The book will offer insights on building meaningful connections, understanding different perspectives, and adapting your communication style to create a sense of trust and collaboration.

- **Overcoming Resistance and Objections**: The book will provide strategies to address skepticism, handle objections effectively, and anticipate potential challenges.

- **Ethical Considerations**: The book will emphasize the importance of ethical persuasion and provide guidelines on maintaining integrity, respect, and empathy.

So, let's get right into becoming more persuasive with 10 simple hacks!

Chapter 1: Building Rapport

When two or more people feel mutually coordinated, positive to one another, and trust each other, they experience rapport (Brown, 2022). This will help you in your profession when you engage with customers, but also in your social life for establishing a strong network.

Do you wish you could make a meaningful, almost instant connection with your audience? In this chapter, we'll explore techniques that will allow you precisely that!

Create a Sense of Familiarity

When somebody finds themselves speaking to another person who somehow resembles them, they tend to open up and feel more comfortable. Here are some ways in which you can create a strong first impression with a potential customer or a new acquaintance that will make them feel an almost instant rapport.

Mirror Body Language

Most of our communication is non-verbal, and the way we use our gestures, posture, and facial expressions transmits more than we think. When you engage in a conversation, try noticing the small gestures of the other person—if they cross their legs, scratch their nose, or casually take a sip of water after making a statement. You don't want to fully imitate them but subtly copy a few of their gestures to create a subconscious connection that will make your speaker feel understood and comfortable around you.

Matching the Pace and Tone of Speech

Your voice is your main tool for communicating. I'm sure you put a lot more attention to your tone, your pronunciation, how you organize your sentences, and other nuances in your speech when you are giving a formal address, don't you? When you are talking to someone, pay attention to how they talk and match that pace. Speaking too fast can leave the impression what you say isn't that important, while speaking too slowly may lose your audience's interest.

In the same way, if they tend to speak loud or soft, try adjusting your voice volume to match theirs. As for the tone, it means creating a "music-like" cadence to your speech to avoid sounding monotonous and boring. Speak as if you were reading a punctuated text. Make sure you add inflection to your questions and exclamation marks but still sound natural.

Of course, you'll never imitate the other person's accent, or repeat their speech errors! This is about validating their identity, not mocking them.

Establish a Connection

Find Common Ground

By establishing some common ground—discussing a recent news event, asking them about their weekend, or discussing their music interests—you can create a sense of connectedness that will help you create rapport even if you have just met the person. Politics or religion are controversial topics, so avoid them!

Pay attention to the adjectives the person uses: Do they say something is "great" or "amazing"? Try mirroring them in some parts of the conversation. Again, it's not about imitating them but creating the feeling you both speak the same language.

Likability Through Compliments

When people receive a compliment, this boosts dopamine (a feel-good hormone) in their brains (Brown, 2022). Making a nice comment about your potential customer's hairdo, shirt, or even something positive about the weather will increase the feeling of confidence in themselves. Of course, you can't just praise people expecting something in return; only state compliments if you actually mean them.

The Right Dosage of Humor

You want to make the other person smile so they are more likely to engage with you. Telling them a short, funny story, such as your kid spilling their milk on your papers or you almost missing a bus is the right way to show yourself as vulnerable without losing credibility or looking unprofessional.

Of course, you don't want to be the office clown or crack a joke at the expense of someone you just met. But injecting a little humor into your talk can help you create a light and enjoyable atmosphere. It displays self-confidence and makes you relatable.

Create a Trustworthy Image

People are more likely to comply with requests from someone they know, like, and trust. These are a few ways in which you can increase those feelings right from day one.

Give a Solid First Impression

The way you stand, how you dress, your handshake, and your smile all contribute to creating a strong first impression. If you are shy, try practicing how you introduce yourself in the mirror before meeting someone for the first time. Check out your clothes and your face before you go out there. An unbuttoned shirt or food between your teeth can deeply affect the way people perceive you.

Show Genuine Interest

Smiling and being an active listener both make people trust you. Hold eye contact, nod your head, and avoid distractions (looking at your phone screen). But don't do this for show, being an active listener means you are truly interested in what the other person has to say.

When someone is speaking to you, try to genuinely understand what they are saying. If it's a potential customer, instead of focusing on pitching your product, be open to their needs. Ask them questions and summarize what the other person said in your own words. This not only proves to them you were listening but also makes them feel understood and cared for on a deeper level (Jacoby, 2023).

Use the Reciprocity Principle

When you offer something first, people tend to feel in debt with you which makes them more likely to comply with later requests from your side. This is because it is deeply wired in our human nature to be reciprocal (Hum, 2022). In sales, this could be translated as offering something exclusive and personalized to make the other person feel special and indebted to you. We'll learn more about that in Chapter 6.

Ask for Input

After taking a long speech turn, make sure you ask the other person for their point of view, or if they have any questions. You want to validate them and share an appreciation for their thoughts. Compliment their ideas even if you have to redirect them later: "I think it's an interesting color choice! I believe we could get the same results if we picked this one as well..."

Chapter 2: Anchoring

We like to think of ourselves as logical, purely reasonable people when it comes to decision-making but, the truth is, emotions influence all of us on a deep level and most of the time our emotions and feelings play a big role in the outcome of our decisions. This is true for yourself as well as for others and, knowing that, you can consciously implement certain techniques that will allow you to establish positive emotions and feelings and connect them with the desired actions or outcomes.

What Is Anchoring?

Anchoring is a method of neuro-linguistic programming (NLP) in which a person can trigger a specific emotion or psychological state with a given word, gesture, or other stimulus (Nutley, 2023). Just like the anchor is an element that stabilizes a ship, anchoring associates two experiences together by repetition. Basically, you train yourself or others to link an internal state with something external (Thomas, 2023). You have probably heard about the experiment Ivan Pavlov performed back in the 1920s involving a dog and the sound of a bell, right? Any time the dog was given food, Pavlov rang a bell, to the extent that the mere sound of the bell made the dog drool in anticipation of the delicious treat.

Using Anchors in Others

Advertisers use anchoring all the time. They want their audience to attach positive feelings and impressions to the product they are selling. But no matter what you do for a living, learning some anchoring strategies may come in handy in your daily life.

For example, imagine that you want your toddler to eat their vegetables. A possible anchor would be to play a fun song during dinner every time you prepare a meal they like (pizza?) and then, when you serve them their greens, play that same song to help them associate their plate with that feeling of satisfaction and willingness to finish their food.

Using Anchors in Yourself

You can use anchoring to enhance your self-esteem, elicit a state of calm, or achieve any other useful state that will help you reach your goals. Again, songs work great. Think about how good it feels to train while listening to the *Rocky* soundtrack!

Gestures or words also work. For example, if you want to enhance your confidence, whenever you are feeling particularly proud about yourself pat your right hand with the left one. Do it when someone gives you a compliment, when your spouse smiles at you, or when you see one of your children running towards you after school. Next time you are giving a presentation at work, pat your hand again. Subconsciously, your mind will elicit that same positive sense of accomplishment and pride that will set you right on track for success in front of your boss and colleagues.

Subtle Influences

Different emotions make us prone to viewing certain events from a totally different angle. For example, let's imagine you turn on the TV and see the news about an upcoming strike. Depending on your current mental state, you may perceive it in a completely different way. An angry person may see the negative event as something predictable and controlled by others, while a fearful person may believe the situation is out of control and riskier than it actually is. Turning off the TV and blaming the corporations is not the same as being stressed out of fear you may lose your job.

Learning how powerful emotions can be when it comes to influencing decisions and mental states, you can use subtle cues or triggers to bring back a feeling or reaction—especially if you do it without others noticing. For example, as a manager, you want your employees to feel more comfortable around you. You could use a specific smell, such as some homemade baked goods or fresh coffee grounds, to create a welcoming atmosphere in your office that reminds people of home.

Or, if you always use a calm, confident tone of voice when saying something nice to your partner, and then you replicate the exact same tone when you need to correct them or ask them for something, you'll notice they'll be more receptive to your words, even if it's not something they particularly want to hear. This way, you may avoid them getting defensive.

Retelling the Story

Are you tired of always failing? If you keep telling yourself you are not good at making friends, or that no one in their right mind would hire you, it's no surprise your social life is scarce and you keep getting rejected during your work interviews. You have established a victim's mindset and are living up to it.

Victim or Victor?

So, how can you correct this mindset? The first thing is acknowledging the way you think; you have to stop being a victim and start being a victor. Victims don't take responsibility for their actions and blame others instead while victors have won against the harsh world (Porras, 2022). Stop feeling sorry for yourself. Do something to make a change and become accountable for your own mistakes, instead of looking for someone to blame. Look out for new opportunities and embrace gratefulness for everything you already have. Even in the most difficult situations, you have choices; reclaim that power over your life.

Role Models

Telling the right story is also important for persuading others. Imagine, for example, that your company has lost a major client and your employees feel discouraged. You can tell them about your grandfather, who came to the country with nothing but a suitcase, running away from World War II, and with lots of effort managed to build the business from scratch.

Never underestimate the impact of powerful life stories! Whether you want to sell a product or service, you can inspire people by showcasing relatable role models, evoking in your audience positive emotions such as inspiration and hope.

Chapter 3: Social Proof

No matter how much we struggle to be one-of-a-kind and have authentic, unique opinions, all of us are sensitive to what other people think. Concepts like tendencies, peer pressure, or crowd-pleaser wouldn't exist otherwise. Knowing all that, you can apply certain psychological tools to make your content socially compliant. Let's explore them!

What Is Social Proof?

With social proof, we mean a psychological phenomenon in which people tend to copy or consider the actions of others to establish the right way to behave. For example, if you were walking down the street and you noticed everyone around you was suddenly rushing the opposite way, you'd probably change your course without even asking what's wrong, as you'd assume there is a danger somewhere ahead.

Marketing and advertising industries use social proof all the time as a way of boosting their effectiveness in selling products or services. There are six main types of social proof (Lua, 2017):

- **Expert**: If a doctor recommends a specific vitamin supplement, it must be good because they have studied medicine and therefore, they know better.

- **Certification**: Similar to the expert, here the social proof comes from a stamp by an authoritative figure (for example, if a didactic toy has the approval of the American Academy of Pediatrics or AAP).

- **Celebrity**: When celebrities endorse specific products, people are attracted to those brands because they want to be just like that celebrity.

- **User**: The recommendation of someone who is currently going to a gym in your neighborhood is more likely to get you to join the same gym. After all, they have experienced it and you haven't.

- **The crowd**: If a brand is the favorite of millions, you are more likely to try it. One would guess they can't *all* be wrong, can they?

- **Your friends**: When you see a friend using a product or following a brand on social media, you are more likely to use it yourself.

Highlighting Popularity, Endorsements, or Testimonials

Knowing what social proof is, you can design your communication strategy using testimonials of others to create a sense of social validation and encourage compliance. If you are designing a campaign for your social media, try inviting an expert to endorse your service or product. You can offer mutual collaboration, or find someone who actually likes what you sell and is willing to share their opinion with the world. If you manage to get a celebrity that works just as well! Besides that, sharing great reviews from your customers, or offering "success stories" as part of your content also helps.

However, don't feel tempted to implement all the tactics at the same time. According to Ali, it's better to "select 2-4 kinds that make the most sense for your business, and put together a plan to implement them over the next 3-6 months" (2023).

Another example of social proof, this time outside business: If your mother-in-law won't listen to you when you specifically told her you don't want to feed anything to your two-month-old other than breastmilk, let her know that the AAP recommends exclusive breastfeeding up to six months. She'll probably think twice before sneaking that cookie to your baby!

Alignment With Beliefs or Previous Commitments

We naturally have an inner desire to align our actions with our beliefs or previous commitments because we strive for consistency. If a brand aligns with a specific value, *not* choosing that brand would subconsciously mean that you are *not* following that value. People don't want to feel inconsistent in their behavior, so the stronger they align with a brand's belief, the more likely they are to choose it. So if you manage to link your brand with a certain value, you are likely to catch the attention of people who follow that value.

For instance, you state that sustainability and waste reduction are essential parts of taking care of the environment, and you appeal to people who believe in making a change. When later you state that the line of reusable cups you produce creates less waste than other brands, people who share the environmental cause are more prone to buying your product. Encourage your audience to align their actions with their existing beliefs or commitments, making it harder for them to contradict themselves.

Group Acceptance

Whether consciously or not, to some degree people tend to follow the leader. No wonder why popular opinions are—you know—popular! If you manage to demonstrate that lots of people are already choosing your product or service, others are more likely to take the desired action as well. Making it public when you reach important numbers of followers, for example, will make you gain new ones in the blink of an eye.

We're even more influenced by this principle if we are insecure about ourselves, or if we perceive the people we observe are similar to us in some way (Schenker, 2022). That's why social media targets their advertising campaigns to specific groups; working moms aged 30-45, teenagers on the West Coast, or retired senior citizens, to name a few.

How would this work in real-life persuasion? We use it all the time without realizing it! Or hasn't your teenage daughter ever mentioned that "all the other parents" were allowing their kids to attend a certain party? If that didn't change your mind, at least it made you hesitate, as you too want to be perceived as part of the "cool parents" group. Am I wrong?

Chapter 4: Scarcity

Perhaps you've seen it in a playground: The swings are empty until a couple of kids go to play on them. In a matter of seconds, every child in the park can't wait to get on a swing and they form a long line and throw the occasional tantrum. It's not just because they are kids. Remember March 2020, when supermarkets all across the US ran out of toilet paper because people started to hoard the packages as if their lives depended on them?

It's part of human nature. When people perceive that something is limited or in short supply, this creates a sense of limit and urgency and moves them to act. Due to its scarcity, the value of something rises, even when it wasn't perceived as a necessity before. Let's see how we can implement strategies to take advantage of this technique.

Definition of Scarcity

Scarcity is the perception that something is unique, rare, and only available for a selected few. It doesn't necessarily have to do with the current number of products available. Again, it's a matter of *perception*. Thinking of a purse as "exclusive" makes it more valuable, even if there are ten thousand copies of the same model of the purse. And when an item becomes demanded by more people, its price rises.

The concept of scarcity is related to the one of urgency, although they aren't exactly the same. Urgency refers to time. When people perceive that something is time-sensitive, about to expire, or to change, they act out quickly because they develop a sense of fear of missing out or FOMO. Just think about how so many people go crazy on Black Friday, and how many of those purchases are impulsive—and sometimes unnecessary!

In any case, scarcity and urgency work in creating in potential customers an emotional response that makes them prone to acting, and therefore, these techniques are widely implemented in pricing strategies.

Create a Perception of Limited Availability or Time Sensitivity

So, how can you apply these principles to persuade your audience? In marketing or advertising, when you present your product as a limited, time-sensitive, numbered stock, or limited-edition item, it can create a sense of scarcity. Let's imagine you are advertising your professional hair braiding salon on social media: You could mention a last-minute offer due to a cancellation, hairstyles at half price for the first three people to answer the ad. Of course, there wasn't any cancellation and you just happened to have the afternoon available, so you are not losing money but actually gaining a few new customers for that day that are likely to return some other time.

Another way is announcing your prices are going to rise soon, and this is the last chance for your customers to book an appointment with the former price. The perception of time limitation works just as well.

If you are selling products instead of services, labeling some of them as "exclusive", "time-limited edition", "limited stock", or one-of-a-kind items makes the audience perceive your product as prestigious and increases its perceived value and demand. For example, if you are releasing a new model of reusable diapers, you could create a campaign announcing that one of their designs is only available for the first 20 buyers.

You can also create a sense of scarcity with services. A common strategy implemented by luxury brands is having the service available only through invites or recommendations from previous users. This also gives the service social proof—as seen in Chapter 3—since it creates in potential users the idea that they get to "belong" to a selected few. By emphasizing scarcity, you can increase the perceived value of whatever you are offering. When people believe something is scarce, they tend to assign a higher value and feel a sense of urgency to acquire it before it becomes unavailable.

Can you implement the scarcity principle to persuade people in your daily life? Sure! Again, it works by creating a sense of limitation and urgency. For example, your four kids are lazying around on the couch and your hands are full with dinner preparation. You could casually mention you only have one Kit-Kat and it's for whomever sets the table (although you'll probably have to split the candy bar in four).

The Fear of Missing Out (FOMO)

Scarcity enhances the fear of missing out or FOMO, which is the anxiety people experience when they feel they will miss out on something valuable or exciting. It's a powerful motivator that makes you act quickly because you are scared that otherwise you'll be left out.

FOMO is a rather new term, as it was first introduced in 2004 in direct relation to social networking sites: "FoMO includes two processes; firstly, perception of missing out, followed up with a compulsive behavior to maintain these social connections" (Gupta & Sharma, 2021). Social media enhances FOMO through resources such as Instagram stories, which are only available for 24 hours and thus, make users promptly click on them before they disappear.

Although FOMO has been linked with negative effects on mental health (because it creates emotional tension, lack of sleep, and when it comes to social media, can replace face-to-face interactions), it can also be used as a motivation for good purposes. For example, holding a streak in a learning app like Duolingo maintains your motivation for staying on a language course and keep on learning.

Although it's a good idea to implement the strategy of scarcity in marketing, don't overdo it. You want your potential customers to appreciate the uniqueness of your product or service, not to see your brand as manipulative.

Chapter 5: Authority

Back in Chapter 3, we've already mentioned a kind of social proof that comes from being endorsed by an expert. What if you *are* the expert? Then, your audience will believe you and feel more inclined to follow you. Let's see some ways in which you can create a sense of authority and expertise—notwithstanding your lack of official credentials!

Establishing Expertise and Credibility

If people are going to invest time, money, energy, or enthusiasm with somebody, they want to do so with someone they can trust. This works both in the corporate world as well in daily life situations. In any case, part of persuading your audience is establishing your expertise and credibility through knowledge, credentials, or endorsements to enhance your persuasive influence.

Some steps are essential for building credibility:

- **Be professional**: Display an appropriate look and keep your emotions under control. Don't take criticism personally, and never attack a person, only the flaws in their arguments.

- **Be transparent and authentic**: Be open and honest about your intentions. If you are looking to make a sale, it's because it's beneficial both to you and your customers.

- **Be an expert**: Know your product and service. You must be ready to promptly address any questions or concerns. Don't run the risk of giving wrong information or guiding someone into a bad decision because you're not up-to-date with your knowledge.

- **Be sensitive**: You may be a true authority in the field, but if you fail to empathize with your audience and forget to display humbleness about your accomplishments, you will sound arrogant, and no matter how much authority you display, it won't help you persuade them.

The Tendency to Comply with Experts

According to the principle authority in social psychology, people naturally comply with experts or authorities in a particular field. We perceive that people in a position of authority have greater wisdom and power, therefore, we're more likely to obey them. For example, if your spouse suggests you put less salt in your meals because it's terrible for your health, you may disregard their well-intentioned advice. But would you do the same if the person who said it was a doctor?

Blind authority and obedience have a dark side as well, as was demonstrated during the Milgram experiment, in which a group of subjects was asked by a scientist to administer electrical shocks to another person (who was actually a confederate of the researchers). Despite thinking the other person was in pain, or even in danger, most of the test subjects still obeyed the orders of the authorities (Fessenden, 2018).

That's why being an authority has ethical implications. Knowing about your field doesn't mean you should misguide your audience or deceive your potential customers under false pretenses. On the other hand, it means that you have the power to guide them through making a conscious, informed decision backed by your expertise.

The same applies in your relationships: You want your children to obey you because you, the adult, know what's best for them. Explaining to them the consequences of their decisions and telling them about your life experience is very different than simply stating they have to listen to you "because I say so."

Establishing Trust

People tend to trust people they perceive as authorities. They are more receptive to their messages and ideas. You can influence your employees, your potential customers, or any audience if you can establish a sense of trust. Besides showing off your credentials, you need to become a reliable person.

In the workplace, you need to make sure your staff knows you're on their side. You will project an image of confidence and trust by being consistent (doing what you say you'll do and keeping your promises), being open and friendly, admitting your own mistakes, showing support to your team when they inevitably make theirs, and respecting other people's perspectives.

Unfortunately, building trust takes a lot of time and effort, and all of it can be lost in a matter of seconds. Once you've lost trust, it's really hard to recover it. That's why you need to make sure your words match your actions every single time, and not just most of the time. Think about how it works in friendships or in marriage: You may have been loyal for years, but if you betray someone even once, you may lose the friend or break the marriage for good.

Demonstrating Knowledge and Expertise

To gain credibility and influence, you must present yourself as an expert in your field. You can demonstrate your expertise by sharing valuable insights, providing accurate and up-to-date information, and deeply understanding the subject matter. By showcasing your expertise, you enhance your persuasive power and establish yourself as a go-to source in your area of specialization way more than just by hanging a diploma on your office walls or displaying a seal of approval in your packaging.

Also, while having a college degree or a credential in your area of expertise is great for establishing authority, it's not enough. You also need to show you are always willing to learn and keep your knowledge up-to-date. Besides, not all of our expertise comes from books and courses, as most of our knowledge comes from experience.

In that sense, asking questions, listening to others, and accepting constructive feedback don't undermine your credibility, quite the contrary! According to Schooley, willingness to learn new skills is among the most crucial qualities employers look for when hiring new team members (2023).

Even if you are an expert in your field, being open to suggestions, new ideas, or constructive criticism will increase your expertise and keep alive both an impression of authority as well as certain flexibility and openness to new challenges.

Chapter 6: Reciprocity

Part of living in a society is knowing how and when to exchange things or favors with others to gain a mutual benefit. People are more likely to help you if they feel like they "owe you" because you did something nice first. If you welcome your new neighbor with a basket full of fresh-grown vegetables from your garden, they are likely to say yes when you later require a favor from them, such as watering your plants while you are on vacation.

The rule of reciprocity is a social norm, which means it's not necessarily stated formally, but somehow has become a habit that allowed us to build communities and achieve more together than we could have ever dreamed of if we were by ourselves. In this chapter, we'll explore how to use reciprocity as a persuasion technique.

The Concept of Reciprocity

The need to reciprocate comes from the early development of social skills. Even when we are toddlers we learn how to share or take turns since these are important skills for living among others. It is vital both for establishing and maintaining relationships. If you are the only one who always calls your friend and suggests seeing each other, or if you remember their birthday but they keep forgetting yours, or if you ask them about their health but they never care about you, then that friendship is not meant to last.

However, reciprocity doesn't only involve personal favors or tangible objects but plays an important role in influencing and persuading others to follow your beliefs and obey your commands.

Applying Reciprocity for Persuasion

Give Something of Value First

Together with other concepts already explored, such as social proof or authority, reciprocity is one of Dr. Robert B. Cialdini's principles of persuasion. Simply put, you aren't only inclined to pay back a favor, you are wired to feel obliged to do so. This way, if you begin by giving your audience something that's good for them, they'll feel the urge to give you something in return (Schenker, 2022).

How does this work in marketing or sales? One effective way is by offering value to others before asking for compliance. For instance, let's say you want to sell homemade pies and cupcakes online. Instead of simply displaying them and advertising them, you could include in your website free baking recipes or advice. This would make your visitors prone to buying your products, as they have already got something from you.

Providing something meaningful, such as resources, creates a sense of indebtedness in the recipient. This increases the likelihood that they will feel obligated to reciprocate the favor. Free samples or discounts work the same way.

Use Positive Affirmations

Positive affirmations can be crucial in creating reciprocity. Acknowledging behaviors that lead in a desired direction is the best way to keep them going. For example, if you want to persuade your partner it is time to move to a new house, you could begin your conversation by thanking them for taking the time to consider it in the first place. Other examples of positive affirmations are the following:

- I like how you handled the situation.
- I couldn't have managed so well if I were you.
- That's a great suggestion!
- You clearly understand my point of view.

By using language that reinforces positive beliefs and encourages others to imagine the desired outcome, you can make people feel more inclined to reciprocate your actions. However, for it to work, your affirmations must be genuine and coherent. You can't praise a suggestion and totally dismiss it immediately afterward.

Incorporate Visual Elements

Around 65 percent of human beings are visual learners, which means they acquire information faster through visuals than text only (*5 reasons to use visual aids*, 2021). And when people can visualize the benefits they will receive or the impact of their compliance, they are more likely to reciprocate.

Visuals grab and maintain your audience's attention for longer and also make them better at retaining important concepts. This is especially important during long presentations. At the same time, visualizing your ideas makes them easily understood and helps you establish an emotional bridge between you and your audience, making them more compelled to care about what you're saying.

Visual aids, such as charts or slides, can enhance engagement. Using visual elements to convey information can make your message more compelling and memorable. This doesn't necessarily mean you'll persuade your audience, but it definitely increases your chances.

Offer Some Kindness

We've seen how reciprocity is deeply ingrained in human nature. By offering something meaningful to others, such as a gift, a favor, or a kind gesture, you tap into this innate desire to give back.

During the 2020 Covid pandemic, many brands offered free products or services for essential workers, such as NHS staff. Some others—such as fitness or educational brands—provided free online classes or courses for all the family. Many brands also reshaped their logos or slogans to encourage social distancing.

Despite none of these measures being aimed at an immediate economic gain, reciprocity helped them emerge stronger than ever: "These brands have displayed wonderful acts of kindness during a global crisis, and in the long term these brands and celebrities will inevitably be thought of favorably and will no doubt reap the rewards" (Leonard-Myers, 2020).

You don't need a new global crisis to apply the same strategy. Promoting good causes or donating to charity can do wonders for your brand, even if you don't obtain a direct profit in return.

The Desire to Give Back

Reciprocity works in your daily life and your personal relationships as well, driven by that human instinct to give back when someone has provided to us or done us a favor. If you are a good listener, do a favor, or are willing to make a commitment, the other person will feel the desire to balance the scales of give-and-take.

For example, in a healthy marriage, reciprocity means both participants are equally willing to invest in the relationship and that both of them take responsibility for their actions. This doesn't work if you only do nice things for your partner hoping to achieve something in return. By no means should reciprocity be used as a means of control or manipulation.

Chapter 7: Framing and Priming

Imagine you were looking for a hotel and you see one advert with pictures full of candlelight dinners and champagne bottles, and another advert with a happy kid going down the water slide and a happy couple walking down the beach with a couple of toddlers in their arms. Which hotel would you choose? The answer depends on whether you're looking forward to a romantic getaway or a family vacation, of course.

In this chapter, we'll see how you can apply specific strategies to enhance your audience targeting and get a positive response, and how to position your content for maximum impact.

What Are Framing and Priming?

When it comes to marketing, reaching a large number of potential customers is important, but even more important is reaching the right target audience; those who are more likely to react. Thus, you want to elicit a positive emotional response in them. Your efforts should be based on presenting your request or idea in a way that aligns with the individual's existing beliefs to increase receptiveness.

The framing strategy refers to the fact that everybody perceives information in two ways: They consider the costs and benefits of any new situation or purchase. You want to convey your message in a way that highlights the advantages of your product while overshadowing the losses. For example, if you are selling a brand of reusable diapers that are made of a great fabric but are more expensive than other brands, you would highlight the importance of good quality and how long they will last.

On the other hand, priming refers to the strategy of appealing to the subconscious of the audience by triggering positive memories in their minds. It is usually achieved through storytelling. In the aforementioned example of reusable diapers, you could include lovely videos of parents taking care of beautiful, smiley babies, which will be relatable for the customer and will be associated with your brand.

As you can see, both strategies work by creating positive responses toward your brand, although framing appeals more to reason while priming appeals more to emotions.

Align With Existing Beliefs or Positive Framing

When presenting your idea, consider the beliefs and values of your audience. Frame your content to align with their existing beliefs, increasing receptiveness. For example, if you want to sell insurance policies, you want to highlight values such as keeping the family safe, being in control even in unexpected situations (such as needing surgery), or safeguarding lifelong savings.

Framing emphasizes benefits and positive outcomes. Because people are motivated by personal benefits and positive change, by focusing on potential benefits your content becomes more appealing and persuasive. Communicate the value proposition and how your proposal addresses needs. In the same example, while nobody actually enjoys spending money on insurance, as they don't get to see an immediate profit, positive framing highlighting benefits, improves the perception and boosts acceptance. For example, by investing in the right insurance policy, you feel safer, you are protecting your family, you are prepared for the unexpected, and you won't be caught off guard.

Framing can also be applied in everyday communication examples. Let's say you are a teacher and you are planning a school trip that is a bit pricey for your district. You could implement framing for persuading your principal to advocate for the trip while presenting specific content the children will learn during the trip and even figures of how the average grades of the class will increase based on the benefits of such an experience.

Tailor Your Approach

There are many different ways to convey the same message, that's why you need to adapt to your audience's preferences and communication style. You wouldn't use the same advertising campaign if you were targeting teens than if your audience were senior citizens, even if you are trying to sell them something similar (for example, sunglasses). In the same way, you wouldn't ask your five-year-old to help you set the table the same way you'd ask your spouse.

The first thing you need is to know your audience: Who are you communicating with? What are their values? What do they care about the most? A teen looking for sunglasses may want to look cool, while a man in his sixties may want to be able to drive without the sun affecting his vision.

Customize your content to engage them effectively, considering tones and channels. For example, if you are targeting teens you won't spend money on a campaign on Facebook, but rather on TikTok. And your language would be more informal than if you were addressing adults. You need to adjust your language to resonate with your target audience, maximizing your impact.

Identify and Prioritize Core Values

Core values are the attributes each person considers more important than anything in the world. For example, a person may feel their core value is their health. Another may feel it's seizing the day. Core values are also those traits people would like to be known for, such as honesty, kindness, compassion, or intelligence.

In any case, aligning actions with core values is crucial. As a communicator, you should help individuals identify and prioritize their values, guiding their decision-making. For example, in the case of choosing a hotel, core values could be family, enjoyment, safety, and seizing the day (if you want to address parents trying to book a stay for a family vacation), or luxury, intimacy, and relaxation (if you want to address people going on their honeymoon).

When you communicate your idea, you can use priming to emphasize how your content aligns with your audience's values and contributes to personal fulfillment. This connection increases influence and encourages action.

Chapter 8: Using Persuasive Language

Language goes way beyond using words and sentences. We also communicate through our posture, the tone of our voice, and our facial expressions. How can we make sure we're using the best possible tools we have to properly convey our messages and make our audience more receptive and likely to comply with our requests?

Using Persuasive Body Language

Our body is an essential tool for communication. Through our body language, we're constantly sending all kinds of messages, sometimes even without realizing it. And if we want to be persuasive, we need to make sure our body language matches our words. For example, if you tell someone you're happy to see them while keeping a frown on your face, you will sound dishonest: "When faced with such mixed signals, the listener has to choose whether to believe your verbal or nonverbal message. Since body language is a natural, unconscious language that broadcasts your true feelings and intentions, they'll likely choose the nonverbal message" (Segal et al., 2023).

When you are speaking to someone, they will react to the way in which you stand, so you want to project a stable presence. Stand with your feet apart at armpit width and move purposefully (don't just wander around). You should use gestures to emphasize important points in your speech, but make it clean and limited. On the other hand, if you are sitting down when talking (for instance, during a work interview), pay attention to your position: Don't get too comfortable leaning back in your chair, sit up and lean forward. Also, don't cross your arms, as it creates a physical barrier between you and your speaker (Genard, 2013).

Pay attention to the proximity in which you stand when you are talking to someone. The need for physical space is cultural, but invading another person's space will make you seem more intimidating than persuading. Another important factor is eye contact. It is vital for maintaining a conversation flowing because it shows honesty, plus a genuine interest in what your speaker has to say.

Remember how we mentioned how audiences respond to visuals? Well, your body language is the greatest visual element of all, and its importance even predates speech, so you'd better make good use of this powerful resource.

And once you've worked on your abilities to manage your own body language, you'll also start noticing other people's non-verbal cues. Evaluate their tone of voice, eye contact, physical touch (or lack of it), facial expressions, posture, and gestures as a whole. What are they really trying to say? Pay attention to their inconsistencies in case their non-verbal communication contradicts their words.

How to Talk in an Effective Language

Clarity Goes First...

You want to convey your message in a clear, concise way. Your message may be good and strong, but unless you manage to convey it in a way that your audience pays attention to it, understands it, accepts it, and incorporates it into their self-concept, it won't be effective (Jhangiani & Tarry, 2014). That's why most of the time you need plain language, avoiding jargon and acronyms that act as barriers for people who are not familiar with them.

While using jargon (which means words that are specific to a certain group, field, or profession) may work when addressing such a specific target, when you want to persuade a large audience you need to make sure they all understand. Make your message accessible and straightforward. This will increase the chances of acceptance.

Here are some more tips for language clarity:

- Use a logical structure and organization.
- Divide your text into short, simple sentences and paragraphs.
- Choose active voice over passive voice.
- Use personal pronouns and transition words to clarify the relationship between ideas.
- If you need to explain a difficult concept, use examples and analogies to further illustrate it.

Additionally, getting feedback from your audience is a great way for them to tell they understand your message.

...But Subtlety Goes a Long Way

When it comes to advertising, language strategies are different. Sometimes, you don't just go around telling people to book your services right away or buy your product. Instead, you want to subtly influence others' thinking and behavior by directing attention toward a specific action or idea.

Incorporate subtle commands to shape perception and response. For example, instead of using the more aggressive "Book your appointment now" you may implement scarcity and urgency tactics as seen in Chapter 4, and use "Special price for the next 24 hours". Remember to use these patterns ethically and respect individual consent.

At the same time, you want to make sure you acknowledge and appreciate contributions. Recognizing others' efforts has a strong persuasive impact. This is because when people feel valued, they become more receptive to your message. Knowing this, express gratitude and praise to establish rapport and goodwill.

For example, let's say your subordinates are arriving late at the office and you want to make sure they get to work right on time. You should begin your speech by noticing how so many of them are staying after hours to complete their tasks. You appreciate their effort to keep the company's productivity. This will increase your audience's willingness to listen and engage with your ideas. Only then should you introduce the idea that it would be better if everyone arrived right on time for better time management.

Remember that you should model your language according to your specific audience, and that communication goes way beyond words and phrases.

Chapter 9: Harnessing Emotions

Imagine you are feeling the burden of domestic chores is unbalanced at home. You are tired of dealing with all of it. Your spouse loves you but refuses to take the load off your mental burden. What would you rather say to them? "According to a recent survey from FinanceBuzz, you should be paying me at least $15 an hour for domestic chores" (Koebert, 2023), or "I know you love me, but I feel tired and unappreciated when you rely on me for everything"?

When people are looking for reasonable arguments, they may respond to logic, but if you truly want to connect with others and persuade them without them realizing what got them in the first place, you need to appeal to their emotions, as there's nothing more powerful. In this chapter, we'll discuss how to create content to emotionally connect with others.

Harnessing Emotions

Our everyday decisions are influenced by two different parts of our brain: the rational and the emotional. Emotions influence reason far more often than the other way around (Velos, 2021). Advertisers know this well, and that's how they play their cards when it comes to motivating consumers.

By appealing to your audience's emotions instead of using only facts, you will have more influence over them. Emotional feelings are much more likely to foster their loyalty and make them more likely to trust and remember your ad.

Appeal to Emotions Through Storytelling

One of the most powerful techniques to engage your audience emotionally is by telling them a story. Engaging imagination and emotions strengthens the connection, making your content memorable and persuasive. For example, if you want to share the idea that the recipe for your homemade pies is timeless, you could show them the story of a recipe book passing from a lovely grandmother to a young granddaughter on her wedding day.

Use compelling narratives to evoke specific emotions: happiness, anger, fear, and nostalgia. Remember that words aren't as important as visuals. Employ vivid imagery and descriptive language for an emotional experience.

Identify Shared Interests, Experiences, or Beliefs

People don't like being manipulated or being told what to do. Knowing this, when you appeal to emotions you want to create a bond with your audience. You are not here to make them follow you, you are one of them. At the same time, you want to make them feel part of a group, establishing connection and similarity by finding common ground with your audience. When individuals feel understood and reflected in your content, they trust and are influenced by your persuasive efforts.

For example, imagine you want to raise money for a recycling campaign. Through your media content, you should show how you care about the environment and what you are already doing to help. You can also offer free suggestions, such as instructions on how to reuse plastic bottles or how to recycle paper at home. Make sure this content is interactive by inviting your audience to tag your brand in pictures of their own home projects or to share with the community suggestions for reducing waste. Highlight shared interests, experiences, or beliefs that resonate. This creates a bond, increasing receptiveness to your message.

Different Emotions, Different Actions

The different basic human emotions make us respond in different ways. Let's see some of the most common ones (Velos, 2021):

- When people experience sadness, they are more likely to be generous (and therefore, donate to a campaign).

- Campaigns that elicit fear, if well-used, can create a sense of urgency or make people feel more attached to your brand.

- People are influenced by content that makes them feel guilty: For example, a product or treatment to quit smoking that enhances the idea that your children may lose a parent if you carry on with the habit.

- Happiness makes people eager to share, which is why it's a great idea to include it in a campaign or content you want to go viral.

So whether you are looking forward to getting more subscriptions, selling more products or services, following you on social media, or making a donation, appealing to emotions in a deliberate—but by no means manipulative—way, will help the people paying more attention to you, and making your campaign stand out from the thousands of others consumers are exposed to on a daily basis.

Foster Empathy by Understanding Emotions

Your audience already experiences plenty of emotions and perspectives. You want them to feel you understand them and relate to them. Therefore, when you are trying to elicit an emotion to persuade people, first you need to make sure you can actually connect and acknowledge their emotions through empathy.

By empathy, we are referring to the emotional process of putting yourself in the other person's shoes, relating to what they are feeling, their pain points, their worries, and what they are thinking. Listen actively and validate their feelings to show genuine empathy.

For example, imagine you want your mother-in-law to stop dropping by without notice. If you want her to relate to how you're feeling—maybe irritated because of your lack of privacy, possibly embarrassed because she gets to see your house upside down before you have the chance to clean up—start by acknowledging how she must be feeling to act as she does. Maybe she is afraid of losing her only child now that they're no longer living with her, or perhaps she just wants to give the two of you a hand because she felt so lonely when she got married.

In any case, when people feel heard and understood, they become more open to your message. Demonstrating empathy creates meaningful dialogue and strengthens emotional connections.

Chapter 10: Understanding

Resistance and Objections

Whether you are selling a product or trying to convince some of your friends to join you on an adventurous holiday, you are likely to experience some resistance and objections before persuading your audience. In this final chapter, we'll figure out how to best prepare for them.

Resistance as an Emotional Response

Understanding resistance and objections is crucial when persuading someone. We need to understand we are all resistant to change! Imagine you've always disliked cauliflower, and your sister tries to persuade you to try this new recipe she prepared. Although she claims it's delicious, at first your initial response would be "no", right?

When you are the communicator, you need to keep in mind that most resistance is not logical, but emotional (in the example of cauliflower, you may remember experiencing disgust when trying this vegetable for the first time). Therefore, your influence strategy should be based on emotions as well.

The key is encouraging your audience to simply take the first steps. As long as you can move them to give the new experience the chance, they'll realize it isn't as frightening as they thought it would be (Jellison, 2014). That's why test drives, trial runs, free samples, or—when tasting a new dish—taking just a bite, may work like a charm!

Anticipate and Address Objections

Before persuasive conversations, consider potential resistance, which is normal and expected. This works when trying to sell a product or service of any kind. Simply put, if your customers didn't have any objections at all, you wouldn't need to persuade them in the first place! When objections or resistance arise, instead of giving up, you should emphasize the value of your product again. Handling objections can be frustrating, yet it's vital in any sale. How can you do so?

Put yourself in their shoes and actively listen to objections from your potential customers. Only by truly listening to your customer, you'll be able to fully address their concerns. Don't refute them or straight tell them they're wrong! Instead explain why yours is still the best option: "Of course, I understand with our professional babysitting services you'll pay more money than to a teenage girl from the neighborhood. But you should know that if that girl gets sick, you may need to ask for a day off work. This won't happen if you hire professional childcare services".

In a similar manner, empathize with your customer's pain points and offer tailored solutions or compromises: "I see you are uncertain about switching to organic flour. What if I offer you a free sample of the product so you can try a small amount before making an overall change?"

In the end, addressing objections shows understanding and promotes finding common ground for a mutually agreeable outcome.

Encourage Dialogue and Deeper Conversation

Whether you're trying to persuade someone in your personal life or professionally, you must move beyond simple answers by asking thoughtful questions that prompt the other person to express their thoughts and concerns. Use open-ended questions that allow your speaker to explain themselves thoroughly. This fosters a comprehensive understanding of their perspective and enables effective objection handling.

Pushing a customer to buy despite their objections is likely to cause resentment later, or to refrain them from coming back since they perceive you as manipulative. On the other hand, helping your customer make the right choice by addressing their concerns and giving a meaningful response to their objections, is likely to end up with a satisfied customer.

Instead of categorizing any objection as a no, think of them as "speed bumps" that can accelerate leads if you use the right technique (*10 most common sales objections*, 2021). Engaging in meaningful conversation creates an environment for exchanging ideas and finding common ground: "I am aware that our company is relatively new and you may not have heard about us. I can assure you our staff is fully trained and qualified and we can show you their credentials. Additionally, I can give you references from satisfied customers".

Pay Attention, Show Understanding

When people feel heard and understood, they are more open to considering alternative viewpoints and finding common ground. Active listening is crucial for addressing objections. As we explained in previous chapters, it's crucial to attend to both verbal and nonverbal cues. Remember to display your interest through your posture, nodding your head, maintaining eye contact, and avoiding distractions. Use encouraging statements such as "go on" or "I'm listening".

Demonstrate genuine understanding by reflecting on their statements. Paraphrase or summarize what the customer said and validate their concerns. Also, if you later prove them wrong (for example, if their objection comes from misunderstanding or prejudice), showing understanding will prevent any resentment from the customer. For example, "I understand why you think solid shampoo is more expensive than bottled shampoo. You're right, the price tag is actually higher. However, when you consider how long the product lasts on your bathroom shelf, you'll end up saving money in the long run". This validates their perspective and clarifies any misunderstandings.

And even if the customer ends up rejecting your attempts, show gratitude when they refuse. Thank them for their feedback and for the time invested in listening to you. After all, you want to leave them with the best possible impression.

Conclusion

We've seen the importance of a strong communication approach when it comes to conveying a message, both through verbal communication and body language. We've established the importance of active listening, and how understanding and appealing to other people's emotions is key to making yourself understood. Besides, now you know about basic principles of persuasion, such as social proof, scarcity, or reciprocity.

Using the techniques and tips provided in this book, now you are ready to create a call to action for any specific scenario.

Examples

1) **Scenario**: You want to raise money for building shelters for refugees.

   Call to Action: "Join us in making a difference today! By supporting our cause, you can directly impact the lives of those in need. Make your donation now and be a part of positive change."

2) **Scenario**: Your company wants to implement new software and you find resistance among some of your subordinates.

   Call to Action: "Implementing this program can enhance productivity, foster collaboration, and achieve our goals more efficiently. Think of this as an exciting opportunity for us to embrace together!"

3) **Scenario**: Inviting families of your kid's class to attend a Renaissance Fair.

Call to Action: "Come join us! This event promises to bring our community together for an unforgettable experience. Don't miss the opportunity to connect, celebrate, and create lasting memories. Save the date and be a part of something truly special."

4) **Scenario**: Persuading customers to try a new product or service.

Call to Action: "Experience the difference today! Our new product/service offers innovative features to meet your needs. Try it now and unlock a world of convenience, efficiency, and satisfaction."

Being an Ethical Communicator

Remember that persuading does not mean manipulating. Always respect others' boundaries, choices, and well-being, and be mindful of the impact your persuasion attempts may have on them. The responsible and ethical use of these techniques is crucial.

I hope you find the tips helpful and from now on, you find it easier for people to listen and understand your messages, both in your professional and personal life alike!

About the Author

Jayne Watson is an award-winning psychiatric researcher. She received her undergraduate degree from Eastern Oregon State University and her master's from Vasser College. She has been studying mental health issues for over 25 years.

Jayne is passionate about helping to find cures for psychiatric conditions and is an expert on personality disorders and trauma. Understanding the mind of a narcissist became a passion for Jayne when she began a relationship with one. She understands the confusion and pain associated with narcissistic abuse. Jayne teaches what she has learned in her lengthy career so you are armed with the right information to successfully navigate any difficult situation or person.

Your mental health is important for a happy and balanced life. Look for other books by Jayne Watson anywhere best sellers are sold.

References

Ali, H. (2023). *What is social proof, and why is it essential for marketing in 2023?* Wyzowl. https://www.wyzowl.com/social-proof/

Brown, K. (2022). *8 ways to build rapport with clients (professional and fun!).* Science of People. https://www.scienceofpeople.com/build-rapport-with-clients/

Chen, J. (2020, December 18). *Scarcity principle: Definition, importance, and example.* Investopedia. https://www.investopedia.com/terms/s/scarcity-principle.asp

Cherry, K. (2023, March 7). *What is reciprocity?* Very Well Mind. https://www.verywellmind.com/what-is-the-rule-of-reciprocity-2795891

Establishing credibility. (n.d.) Mind Tools. https://www.mindtools.com/aj2ekcx/establishing-credibility. Retrieved on 2023, July 6.

Fessenden, T. (2018, February 4). *The authority principle.* Nielsen Norman Group. https://www.nngroup.com/articles/authority-principle/

5 reasons to use visual aids for speeches and presentations. (2021, July 27). Microsoft. https://www.microsoft.com/en-us/microsoft-365-life-hacks/presentations/five-reasons-to-use-visual-aids-for-speeches-and-presentations

Fryer, B. (2003, June). *Storytelling that moves people.* Harvard Business Review. https://hbr.org/2003/06/storytelling-that-moves-people

Genard, G. (2013, April 21). *Persuade! — How to use body language in a persuasive speech.* The Genard Method. https://www.genardmethod.com/blog/bid/177622/persuade-how-to-use-body-language-in-a-persuasive-speech

Grossman, D. (2022, May 9). *Trust in the workplace: 10 steps to build trust with employees.* The Grossman Group. https://www.yourthoughtpartner.com/blog/bid/59619/leaders-follow-these-6-steps-to-build-trust-with-employees-improve-how-you-re-perceived

Gupta M, Sharma A. *Fear of missing out: A brief overview of origin, theoretical underpinnings and relationship with mental health.* World J Clin Cases. 2021 Jul 6;9(19):4881-4889. doi: 10.12998/wjcc.v9.i19.4881. PMID: 34307542; PMCID: PMC8283615.

Hook, B. (2023, February 26). *How to align with your values.* Values Institute. https://values.institute/how-to-align-with-your-values/

How can you leverage scarcity and urgency to create more demand and value for your product? (n.d.) LinkedIn. https://www.linkedin.com/advice/0/how-can-you-leverage-scarcity-urgency-create-more Retrieved on 2023, July 5.

How do you tailor your communication style to different audiences and channels? (n.d.). LinkedIn. https://www.linkedin.com/advice/3/how-do-you-tailor-your-communication-style-different. Retrieved on 2023, July 7.

How do you use plain language and avoid jargon and acronyms? (n.d.). LinkedIn. https://www.linkedin.com/advice/1/how-do-you-use-plain-language-avoid-jargon-acronyms. Retrieved on 2023, July 7.

Hum, S. (2022, December 15). *6 principles of persuasion to convince anyone to do anything.* Referral Candy. https://www.referralcandy.com/blog/persuasion-marketing-examples

Jacoby, D. (2023, March 24). *How to build rapport in sales with 3 simple techniques.* Sales Readiness Group. https://www.salesreadinessgroup.com/blog/techniques-for-building-sales-relationships

Jellison, J. (2014). *The root of persuasion: How to understand and overcome emotional resistance to be a more effective communicator.* Career Zot. https://ce.uci.edu/careerzot/the-root-of-persuasion-how-to-understand-and-overcome-emotional-resistance-to-be-a-more-effective-communicator/

Jhangiani, R. & Tarry, H. (2014). "Changing attitudes through persuasion" in *Principles of Social Psychology.* Open Text BC. https://opentextbc.ca/socialpsychology/chapter/changing-attitudes-through-persuasion/

Koebert, J. (2023, April 3). *How much is your household labor worth? [Survey].* Finance Buzz. https://financebuzz.com/household-labor-worth-survey

Leonard-Myers, J. (2020, April 9). *The Reciprocity bias, or simple acts of kindness?* The Behaviours Agency. https://thebehavioursagency.com/the-reciprocity-bias/

Lerner, J. S., Li, Y., Valdesolo, P., & Kassam, K. S. (2015). Emotion and Decision Making. *Annual Reviews.* https://doi.org/10.1146/annurev-psych-010213-115043

Lua, A. (2017, May 2). *The psychology of marketing: 18 ways to use social proof to boost your results.* Buffer. https://buffer.com/library/social-proof/

Mirroring body language: The hidden code of connection. (2023, April 11). Become More Compelling. https://www.becomemorecompelling.com/blog/mirroring

Nutley, T. (2023, February 3). *NPL anchoring: A comprehensive guide.* UK College of Personal Development. https://ukcpd.co.uk/nlp-anchoring-a-comprehensive-guide/

Porras, T.M. (2022, December 20). *How do I stop being the victim and start become a victor?* Inspirational Life. https://inspirationalife.com/how-do-i-stop-being-the-victim-and-become-a-victor/

The psychology of emotional and cognitive empathy. (2019). Lesley University. https://lesley.edu/article/the-psychology-of-emotional-and-cognitive-empathy

Quick study guide: Active listening. (n.d.). Devereux. https://learn.devereux.org/nd/guides/qs-Listening.html. Retrieved on 2023, July 10.

Ream, A. (2010, July 12). *Relationships and the importance of reciprocity.* Good Therapy.

https://www.goodtherapy.org/blog/relationship-reciprocity/

Schenker, M. (2022, April 29). *How to use Cialdini's 6 principles of persuasion to boost conversions.* CXL. https://cxl.com/blog/cialdinis-principles-persuasion/

Schooley, S. (2023, February 28). *Career success depends on your willingness to learn.* Business News Daily. https://www.businessnewsdaily.com/9256-career-boost-learning.html

Segal, J., Smith, M, Robinson, L. & Bose, G. (2023). *Nonverbal communication and body language.* Help Guide. https://www.helpguide.org/articles/relationships-communication/nonverbal-communication.htm

10 most common sales objections and how to overcome them? (2021). Deskera Blog. https://www.deskera.com/blog/sales-objections/

Thomas, A. (2023, May 6). *Anchoring.* LinkedIn. https://www.linkedin.com/pulse/anchoring-atnlp/

Vashishtha, H. (2022, April 29). *Priming vs. framing in marketing.* Sixth Factor. https://sixthfactor.com/priming-vs-framing-marketing/

Velos, E. (2021). *How to harness the power of emotion in generating more leads.* Thrive Agency. https://thriveagency.com/news/how-to-harness-the-power-of-emotion-in-generating-more-leads/

Vocal aspects of delivery: Principles of public speaking. (2019). Lumen Learning. https://courses.lumenlearning.com/publicspeakingprinciples/chapter/chapter-12-vocal-aspects-of-delivery/

What are the best ways to evoke emotion in your audience with your content? (n.d.) LinkedIn. https://www.linkedin.com/advice/0/what-best-ways-evoke-emotion-your-audience-content. Retrieved on 2023, July 10.

Ye, L. (2022, December 7). *Objection handling: 44 common sales objections & how to respond.* HubSpot. https://blog.hubspot.com/sales/handling-common-sales-objections